36 Nursing Cheat Sheets
for NursingStudents

NRSNG.com | NursingStudentBooks.com

Jon Haws RN CCRN
Sandra Haws RD CNSC
© TazKai LLC 2015

Introduction

First of all . . . THANKS! Thank you for supporting NRSNG.com and for sharing our mission of improving nursing education. My journey into nursing was a long one but I have found it to be a truly rewarding career that allows me to make a difference and have ample family time. I am confident that you will achieve your goals. The fact that you are seeking additional resources to improve your understanding speaks volumes to your dedication.

The mission of NRSNG.com is to provide you with the confidence and tools you need to succeed . . . in nursing school, on the NCLEX®, and in your life as a nurse!

Second of all, this book is intended to provide you with a quick reference to some of the most needed and most used information for nursing students.

This is not a complete guide to nursing but a simple and compact quick reference to some of the most important information.

As always you should consult institutional policies when it comes to patient care.

Happy Nursing!

-Jon Haws RN CCRN

NRSNG.com | NursingStudentBooks.com

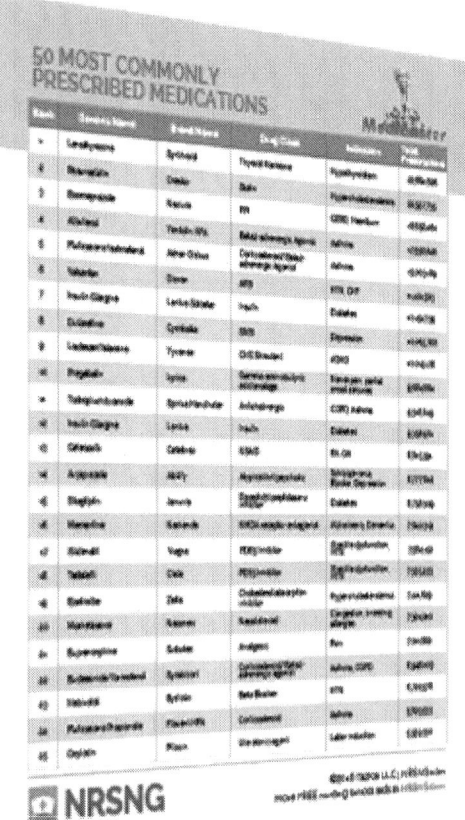

Table of Contents

5 Lead EKG Placement and Heart Sounds

5 Lead EKG Placement & Heart Sounds

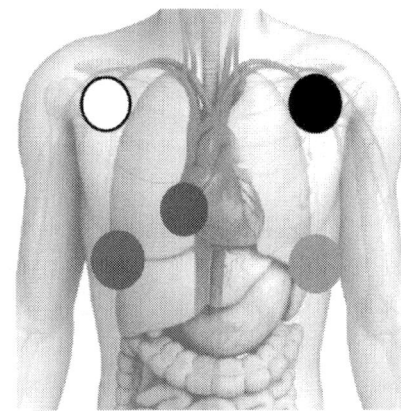

White on Right
Snow over Trees
Smoke over Fire

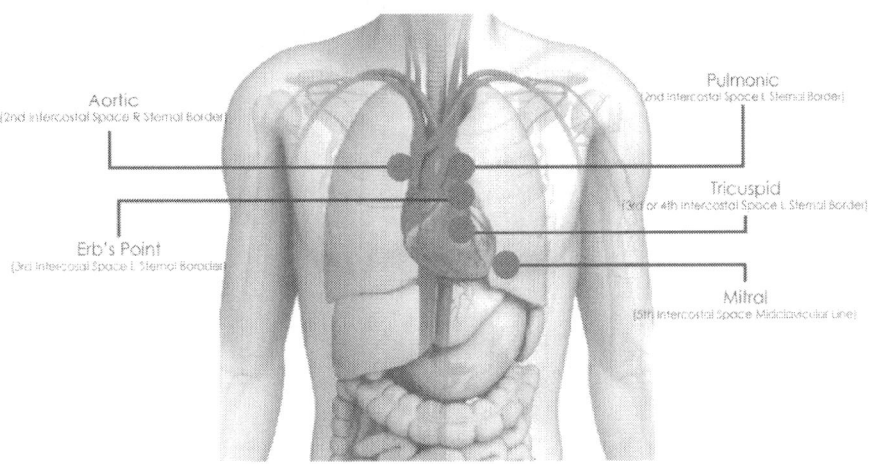

Aortic
(2nd Intercostal Space R Sternal Border)

Pulmonic
(2nd Intercostal Space L Sternal Border)

Tricuspid
(3rd or 4th Intercostal Space L Sternal Border)

Erb's Point
(3rd Intercostal Space L Sternal Border)

Mitral
(5th Intercostal Space Midclavicular Line)

APE To Man
Aortic, Pulmonic, Erbs Point, Tricuspid, Mitral

These locations are optimal for listening to the 4 valves of the heart. Erb's point is the best location to listen for S2. At each location you should listen for any murmur of the associated valve.

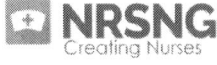

MI Locations and Interventions

12 Lead MI Locations and MI Care

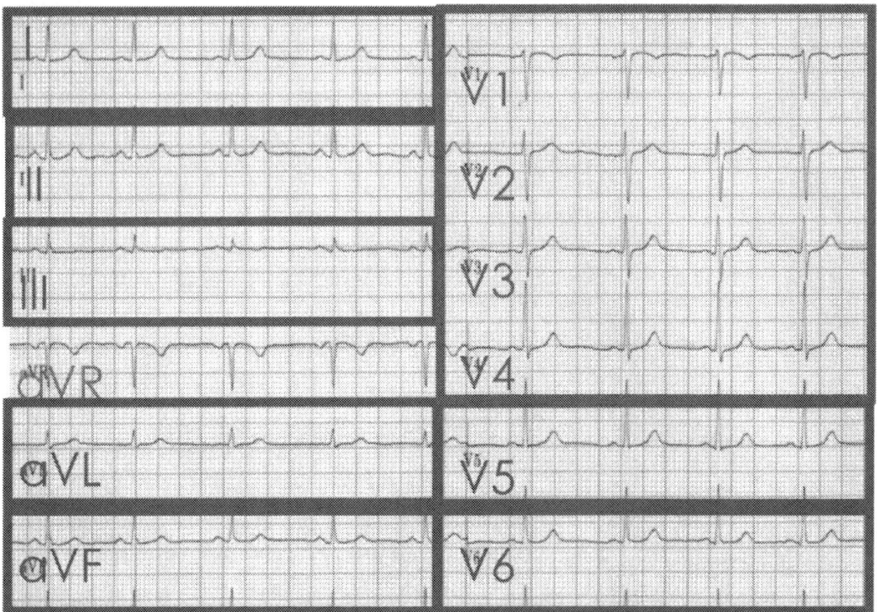

LOCATION	LEADS	ARTERIES
Anterior	V1-V4	LAD
Septal	V1-V2	LAD
Lateral	I, aVL, V5-V6	LCA
Inferior	II, III, aVF	RCA

MI Interventions
M.O.N.A: Morphine, Oxygen, Nitrates, Aspirin

2-4mg morphine q 5-15 minutes
Supplemental O2
0.3-0.4mg nitroglycerine q 4 minutes for 3 doses
160-325mg aspirin

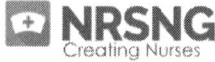

Cardiac Blood Flow and Murmurs

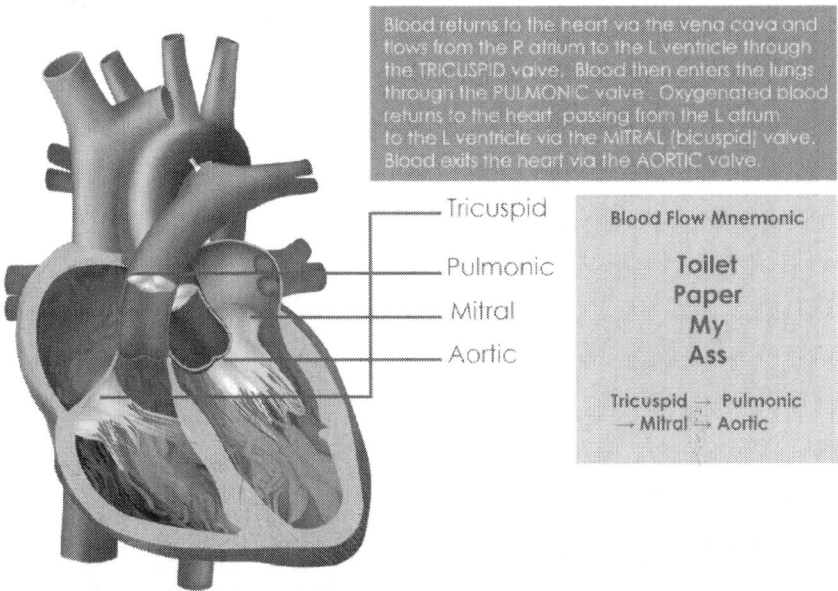

Cardiac Blood Flow and Murmurs

Blood returns to the heart via the vena cava and flows from the R atrium to the L ventricle through the TRICUSPID valve. Blood then enters the lungs through the PULMONIC valve. Oxygenated blood returns to the heart passing from the L atrium to the L ventricle via the MITRAL (bicuspid) valve. Blood exits the heart via the AORTIC valve.

- Tricuspid
- Pulmonic
- Mitral
- Aortic

Blood Flow Mnemonic

Toilet
Paper
My
Ass

Tricuspid → Pulmonic
→ Mitral → Aortic

Heart Murmur Chart

Valve Not Opening = STENOSIS
Valve Not Closing = REGURGITATION

	Diastolic	Systolic
Tricuspid	STENOSIS	REGURGITATION
Pulmonic	REGURGITATION	STENOSIS
Mitral	STENOSIS	REGURGITATION
Aortic	REGURGITATION	STENOSIS

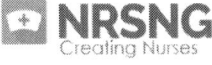

10 Common Heart Rhythms

10 Common Heart Rhythms

NORMAL SINUS	
SINUS BRADYCARDIA	
SINUS TACHYCARDIA	
ATRIAL FIBRILLATION	
ATRIAL FLUTTER	
SUPRAVENTRICULAR TACHYCARDIA	
PREMATURE ATRIAL CONTRACTION	
PREMATURE VENTRICULAR CONTRACTION	
VENTRICULAR TACHYCARDIA	
VENTRICULAR FIBRILLATION	

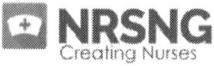 **NRSNG** Creating Nurses ©2016 TazKai LLC | NRSNG.com
More FREE nursing school aids at NRSNG.com
Disclaimer Information at NRSNG.com

Cardiac Labs and Meds

Cardiac Labs and Meds

CARDIAC LABS

Potassium (3.5 - 5)
- Hypokalemia
    - ventricular dysrhythmias
    - ↑ digoxin toxicity
    - U wave
    - ST depression
- Hyperkalemia
    - peaked T waves
    - wide QRS
    - ventricular dysrhythmias

Magnesium (1.5 - 2.5)
- Hypermagnesemia
    - prolonged PR, QRS, QT,
    - brady, blocks
    - cardiopulmonary arrest
    - hypotension
- Hypomagnesemia
    - tachycardia
    - prolonged QT
    - Torsades de Pointes

BNP
- 100-300 HF present
- 300-600 moderate HF
- 600-900 severe HF

↑ Hematocrit (38-50M, 35-45F)
- dehydration

↓ Hematocrit and Hemoglobin
- anemia

Lipids
- Total Chol ↓200 mg/dL
- LDL ↓ 130 mg/dL
- HDL 30-70 mg/dL

COMMON CARDIAC MEDS

Anticoagulants (decrease clotting):
- Heparin
- Warfarin (Coumadin)
- Apixaban (Eliquis)
- Rivaroxaban (Xarelto)

Antiplatelet Agents (clot prevention):
- Asprin
- Clopidogrel (Plavix)

ACE Inhibitors (expand vessels):
- Captopril
- Enalapril
- Lisinopril

ARBS (prevent ACE effects):
- Losartan
- Valsartan

Beta Blockers (decrease CO and HR):
- Metoprolol (Lopressor)
- Propranolol (Inderal)
- Atenolol (Tenormin)

Combined Alpha/Beta Blockers:
- Carvedilol (Coreg)

Ca Channel Blockers (relax vessels):
- Amlodipine (Norvasc)
- Diltiazem (Cardizem)
- Nifedipine (Adalat)
- Nimodipine (Nimotop)
- Nicadipine (Cardene)

Digitalis (positive inotropic effect):
- Digoxin (Lanoxin)

Vasodilators (relax vessels):
- Isosorbide dinitrate (Isodril)
- Hydralazine (Apresoline)
- Nitrates

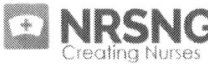 **NRSNG** Creating Nurses ©2016 TazKai LLC | NRSNG.com
More FREE nursing school aids at NRSNG.com
Disclaimer Information at NRSNG.com

EKG Basics and Hyemodynamic Values

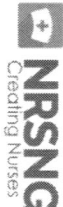

QRS Complex

R

P PR Segment   ST Segment   **T**

PR Interval

Q

S

QT Interval

P wave: 0.08 - 0.10 sec
PR Interval: 0.12 - 0.20 sec
QRS: 0.06 - 0.10 sec

Sinus Rhythm Criteria
Regular rhythm at rate 60-100bpm
Normal P Wave
P Before Each QRS
Constant PR Interval
Normal QRS width

Cardiac Output (CO)		4-8 L/min
Cardiac Index (CI)	CO/BSA	2.5-4 L/min/m²
Cardiac Venous Pressure (CVP)		2-6 mmHg
Mean Arterial Pressure (MAP)	[(2XDBP)+SBP]/3	70-90 mmHg
Stroke Volume (SV)	CO x HR	60-120 mL/beat
Stroke Volume Index (SVI)	SV/BSA	30-65 mL/m²/beat
Pulmonary Artery Occlusion Pressure (PAOP)		8-12 mmHg
Systemic Vascular Resistance (SVR)	80x(MAP-MVP)/CO	800-1400 dynes/sec/cm⁵
Central Venous Oxygen Saturation (ScvO₂)		65-85%
Oxygen Delivery (DO₂)	CO x CaO₂x 10	900-1100 mL/min

O2 Delivery

Heirarchy of O2 Delivery

METHOD

Nasal Cannula
1 lpm = 24%	4 lpm = 36%
2 lpm = 28%	5 lpm = 40%
3 lpm = 32%	6 lpm = 44%

Simple Face Mask
5 lpm = 40%	7 lpm = 50-55%
6 lpm = 45-50%	8 lpm = 55-60%

Non-rebreather Mask
6 lpm = 60%	9 lpm = 90%
7 lpm = 70%	10 lpm = close to 100%
8 lpm = 80%	

Venturi Mask
4 lpm = 24-28%
8 lpm = 35-40%
12 lpm = 50%

Trach Collar
21-70% at 10L

T-Piece
21-100% with flow rate at 2.5 times minute ventilation

CPAP
Positive airway pressure during spontaneous breaths

BI-PAP
Positive pressure during spontaneous breaths and preset pressure to be maintained during expiration

SIMV
Preset Vt and f. Circuit remains open between mandatory breaths so pt can take additional breaths. Ventilator doesn't cycle during spontaneous breaths so Vt varies. Mandatory breaths synchronized so they do not occur during spontaneous breaths.

BI-PAP
Preset Vt and f and inspiratory effort required to assist spontaneous breaths. Delivers control breaths. Cycles additionally if pt inspiratory effort is adequate. Same Vt delivered for spontaneous breaths.

ABNORMAL ABG FINDINGS

	pH	HCO_3	CO_2	Causes
Metabolic Acidosis	↓	↓	↓	DKA, lactic acidosis, diarrhea
Metabolic Alkalosis	↑	↑	↑	vomiting, dehydration, diuretics
Respiratory Acidosis	↓	↑	↑	COPD, CNS depression
Respiratory Alkalosis	↑	↓	↓	CNS d/o, ventilation, hypervent

NORMAL ABG VALUES

pH: 7.35 - 7.45
$PaCO_2$: 35 - 45 mmHg
PaO_2 : 80 - 100 mmHg
HCO_3 : 22 - 26 mEq/L
Base Excess: -2 - +2 mEq/L
SpO_2 : 95 - 100%

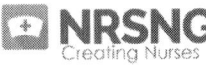

COPD Care

COPD

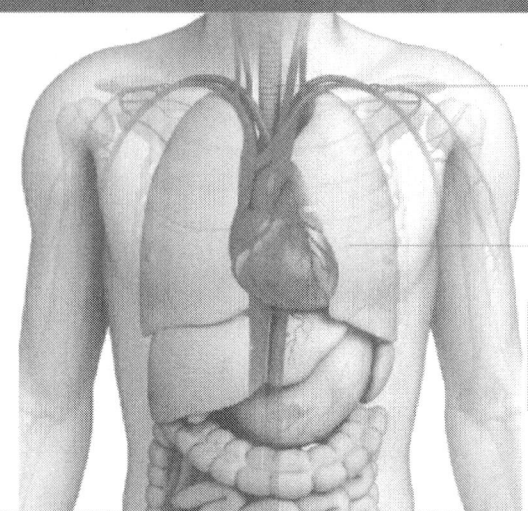

Bronchitis
Inflammation of the lining of the bronchioles with increased mucus.

Emphysema
Destruction of alveoli.

COPD: Progressive obstrucive lung disease characterized by long term poor air flow.

Management of COPD

1. Smoking cessation.
2. Bronchodilators (albuterol, salmeterol).
3. Corticosteroids (fluticasone, budesonide).
4. Phosphodiesterase-4 inhibitor (roflumilast).
5. Antibiotics (prevent frequent resiratory infections).
6. Oxygen therapy (some COPD patient are dependent on hypoxic states for drive to breath as opposed to elevated CO2 as in healthy patient. Assess patient and consult with provider regarding supplemental O2).
7. Activity managment (plan rest with activities).

Neuro Anatomy

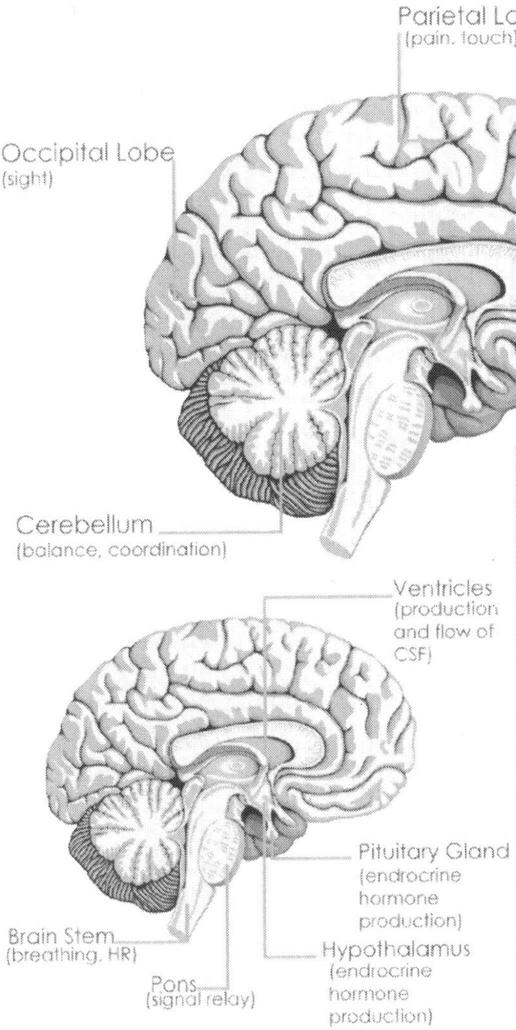

Parietal Lobe
(pain, touch)

Frontal Lobe
(reasoning, planning, speech, movement)

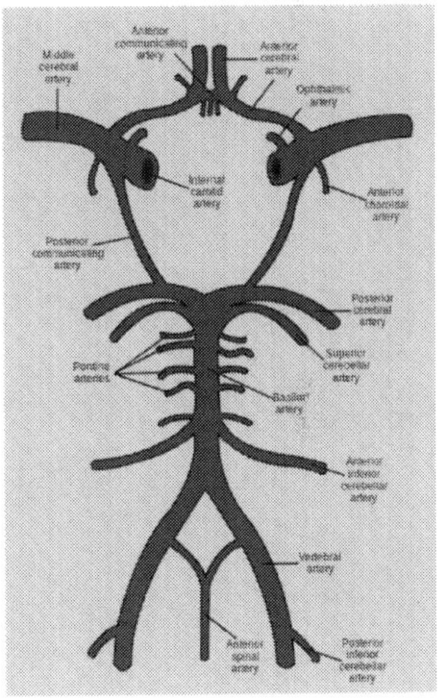

Occipital Lobe
(sight)

Temporal Lobe
(hearing, learning, memory)

Cerebellum
(balance, coordination)

Ventricles
(production and flow of CSF)

Pituitary Gland
(endocrine hormone production)

Brain Stem
(breathing, HR)

Pons
(signal relay)

Hypothalamus
(endocrine hormone production)

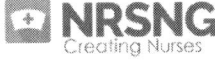

NRSNG
Creating Nurses

NIH Aphasia/Dysarthria

MAMA
TIP-TOP
FIFTY-FIFTY
THANKS
HUCKLEBERRY
BASEBALL PLAYER

You know how.

Down to earth.

I got home from work.

Near the table in the dining room.

They heard him speak on the
radio last night.

Use this sheet to perform steps 9 and 10 of the NIH Stroke Scale.
Resource: http://www.ninds.nih.gov/doctors/NIH_Stroke_Scale.pdf

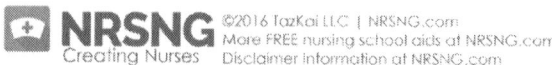

Types of Seizures

Types of Seizures

Focal
- Localized
  - Simple: Remain conscious
  - Complex: Lose consciousness
  - Effects depend on underlying condition

Generalized
- Both Hemispheres
  - Absence (petit mal): lose consciousness <30 sec
  - Myoclonic: <0.1 sec twitch
  - Clonic: repeated "jerking", few seconds - minutes
  - Tonic: muscles contraction lasting <20 sec
  - Tonic-clonic (grand mal): muscle tightening followed by "jerking"
  - Atonic: loss of muscle tone

Status Epilepticus
- No recovery between episodes

Nursing Considerations
- Patient Safety
  - Bed low
  - Turn to side (prevent aspiration)
  - Pad side rails
  - Non-restrictive clothing
  - Prepare to suction
  - Nothing in mouth
- Causes
  - ↑↓ Sodium
  - Medications
  - Fever
  - Drugs
  - Nutrition
- Medications
  - Lorazepam (AED)
  - Fosphenytoin (AED) (check blood levels)
  - Levetiracetam (Benzo)
  - Lacosamide (AED)
  - Midazolam (Benzo)
  - Diazepam (Benzo)
- EEG
  - Aids in diagnosis and managment
- MRI
  - Assess cerebral atrophy and neurological damage

Common Labratory Panels

Common Labratory Panels

Complete Blood Count (CBC)

Value	Abbreviation	Unit	Normal
Red Blood Cell	RBC	x10⁶/mcL	Male: 4.5 - 5.5 Female: 4.0 - 4.9
White Blood Cell	WBC	cells/mcL	4,500 - 10,000
Platelets	PLT	cells/mcL	100,000 - 450,000
Hemoglobin	Hgb	g/dl	Male: 13.5 - 16.5 Female: 12.0 - 15.0
Hematocrit	Hct	Anticholinergic	Male: 41 - 50 Female: 36 - 44
Mean Corpuscular Volume	MCV	fL	80 - 100
Red Cell Distribution Width	RDW	%	<14.5

Basic Metabolic Panel (BMP)

Value	Abbreviation	Unit	Normal
Sodium	Na+	mEq/L	135 - 145
Potassium	K+	mEq/L	3.5 - 5.0
Chloride	Cl-	mEq/L	96 - 108
Glucose	Glu	mg/dL	70 - 115
Calcium	Ca²+	mg/dL	8.4 - 10.2
Creatinine	Cr	mg/dL	0.7 - 1.40
Blood Urea Nitrogen	BUN	mg/dL	7 - 20

Arterial Blood Gas (ABG)

Value	Abbreviation	Unit	Normal
pH	pH		7.35 - 7.45
Partial Pressure of CO_2	$PaCO_2$	mmHg	35 -45
Partial Pressure of O_2	PaO_2	mmHg	80 - 100
Bicarbonate	HCO_3	mEq/L	22 - 26
Base Excess	BE	mEq/L	-2 - +2
Oxygen Saturation	SaO_2	%	95 - 100

Lab Value Skeletons

Lab Value Skeletons

Complete Blood Count (CBC)

WBC   Hct   Hgb   PLT

Liver Enzymes

T. Bili
D. Bili
AST   ALT
ALK Phos

Arterial Blood Gas (ABG)

pH   PaCO2   PaO2   HCO3   SaO2   BE.

Basic Metabolic Panel (BMP or CHEM-7) and CHEM-10

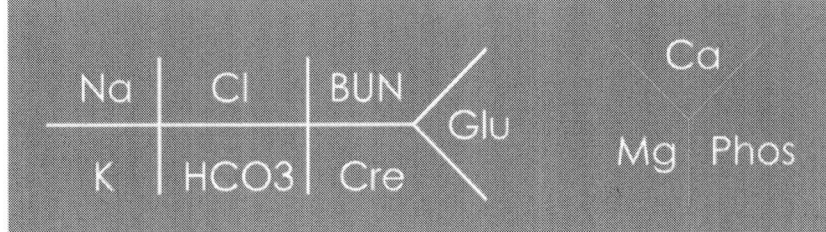

Na | Cl | BUN
K | HCO3 | Cre   Glu

Ca
Mg   Phos

Liver Profile

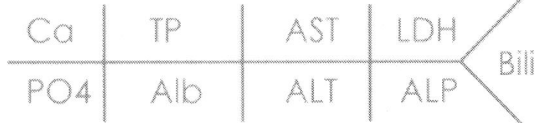

Ca | TP | AST | LDH
PO4 | Alb | ALT | ALP   Bili

Bleeding Times

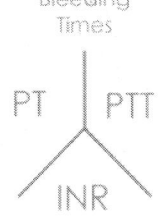

PT | PTT
INR

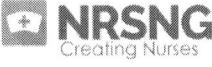

ABG ROME Chart

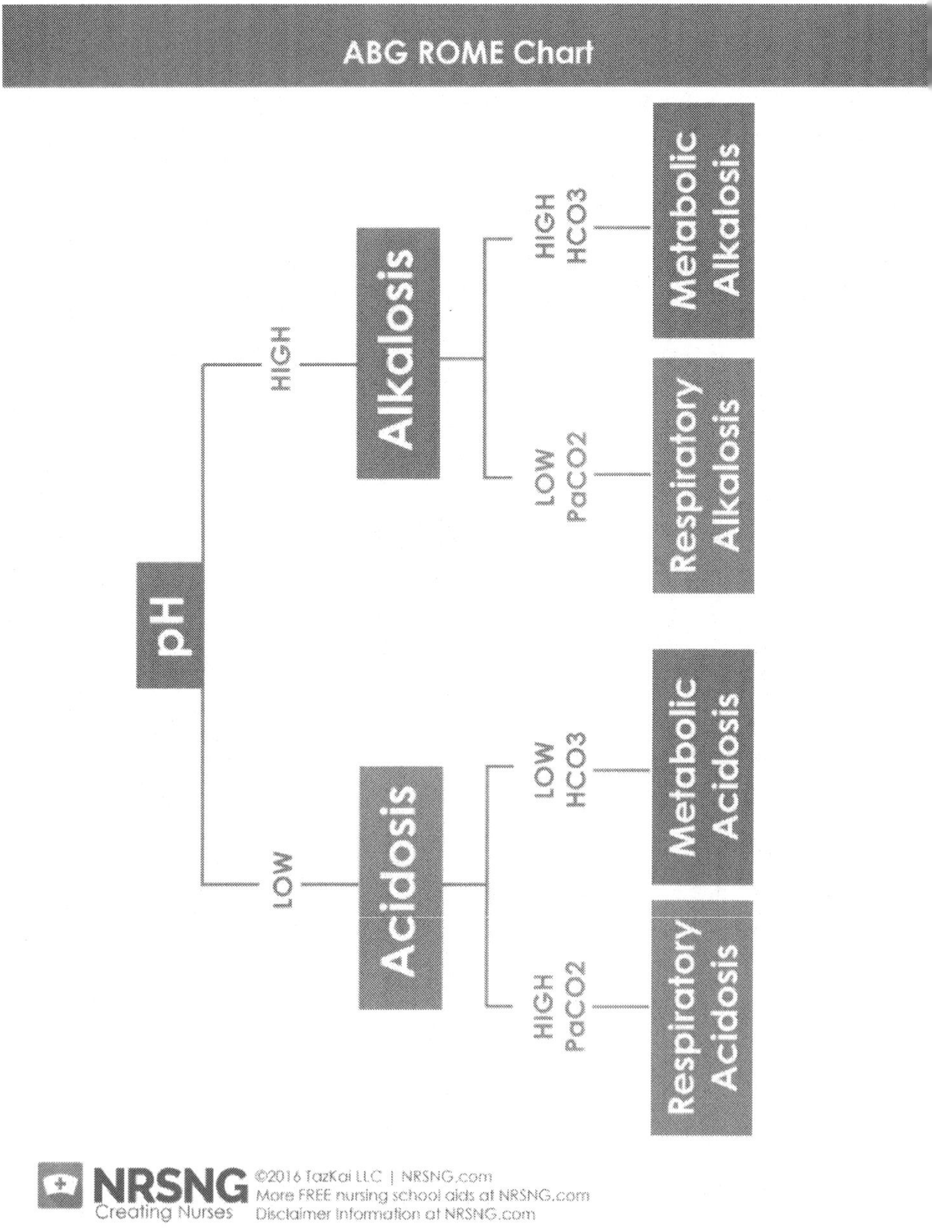

ABG ROME Chart
pH
HIGH
Alkalosis
LOW PaCO2
Respiratory Alkalosis
HIGH HCO3
Metabolic Alkalosis
LOW
Acidosis
HIGH PaCO2
Respiratory Acidosis
LOW HCO3
Metabolic Acidosis
NRSNG
Creating Nurses
©2016 TazKai LLC | NRSNG.com
More FREE nursing school aids at NRSNG.com
Disclaimer Information at NRSNG.com

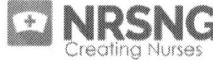

Order of Lab Draws

Order of Lab Draws

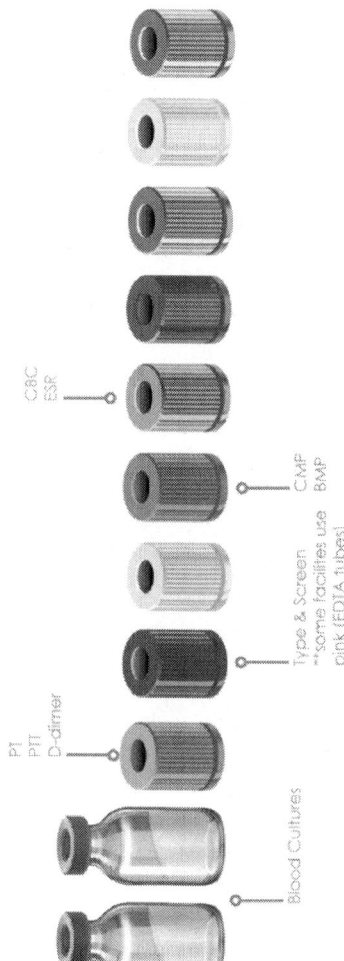

CBC
ESR

CMP
BMP

Type & Screen
**some facilities use
pink (EDTA tubes)

PT
PTT
D-dimer

Blood Cultures

of Times to Invert Tube

Clot Activator - 5 times
Sodium Citrate - 3-4 times
Heparin - 8 times
EDTA - 8 times
Sodium Fluoride - 8 times

Additives by Tube Color

Sterile - SPS
Lt Blue - Sodium Citrate
Plain Red - No Additive
Plastic Red - Clot Activator
Gold, Red/Gray - SST/Gel w/Clot Activator
Green - Heparin-Lithium or Sodium
Lavender, Pink - EDTA
Gray - Sodium Fluoride, Potassium Oxalate

source: http://www.austincc.edu/kotria/phb_tubes and http://96.36.117.186/NewsLetter.pdf
Refer to institutional policies and procedures.

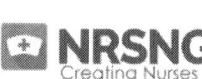

NRSNG
Creating Nurses

Blood Transfusion

Blood Transfusions

PATIENT BLOOD TYPE	DONOR BLOOD TYPE							
	O-	O+	B-	B+	A-	A+	AB-	AB+
AB+	✓	✓	✓	✓	✓	✓	✓	✓
AB-	✓		✓		✓		✓	
A+	✓	✓			✓	✓		
A-	✓				✓			
B+	✓	✓	✓	✓				
B-	✓		✓					
O+	✓	✓						
O-	✓							

Blood Transfusion Reactions

Allergic Reaction
Signs: flushing, itching, rash, hives, fever, edema, swelling

Febrile, non-hemolytic
Signs: chills, fever, palpitations, tachycardia, flushing

Hemolytic
Signs: chills, fever, chest pain, dyspnea, diaphoresis, burning
acute renal failure, flank pain

Sepsis
Signs: chills, very high fever, shock, diarrhea, renal failure

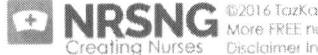 **NRSNG** Creating Nurses ©2016 TazKai LLC | NRSNG.com
More FREE nursing school aids at NRSNG.com
Disclaimer Information at NRSNG.com

Crystalloid IV Solutions

Crystalloid IV Solutions

IVF	Content	Tonicity	Osmolality (mOsm/L)	Uses
D5W	- 50 g/L glucose - 170 Kcals/L - no electrolytes	Isotonic	252	- treat hypernatremia, replace water loss - free water (helps renal excretion of solutes) - used to administer medications
D10W	- 100 g/L glucose - 340 Kcals/L - no electrolytes	Hypertonic	505	- free water only
½NS	- 0.45% saline - 77 mMol/L of Na+ and Cl- - no electrolytes	Hypotonic	154	- maintenance solution, but doesn't replace other daily electrolytes - free water and NaCl - replace hypotonic fluid loss - can cause IVF overload if infused too rapidly
NS	- 0.9% saline - 154 mMol/L of Na+ and Cl- - no calories	Isotonic	308	- used for postoperative fluids - increase IVF and replace ECF fluid losses - NaCl in higher concentration then blood levels - no free water - can cause IVF overload - only solution that can be administered with blood products
3%NS	- 3.0% saline - 513 mMol/L of Na+ and Cl-	Hypertonic	1026	- administer cautiously, slowly treatment for symptomatic hyponatremia - cerebral edema
D5-¼NS	- 0.225% saline - 50 g/L glucose - 170 kcals/L - 38.5 mMol/L of Na+ and Cl-	Isotonic	330	- Provides NaCl and free water - treatment of hypernatremia - replace hypotonic fluid loss
D5-½NS	- 0.45% saline - 50 g/L glucose - 170 kcals/L - 77 mMol/L of Na+ and Cl-	Hypertonic	406	- maintenance solution, but doesn't replace other daily electrolytes - free water and NaCl - replace hypotonic fluid loss - can cause IVF overload if infused too rapidly
D5-NS	- 0.9% saline - 50 g/L glucose - 170 kcals/L - 154 mMol/L of Na+ and Cl-	Hypertonic	560	- increase IVF and replace ECF fluid losses - used for postoperative fluids - NaCl in higher concentration then blood levels - no free water - can cause IVF overload

Medication Prefixes and Suffixes

Medication Prefixes and Suffixes

Prefix/Suffix	Class	Examples
cef-	Cephalosporins (antibiotics)	cefadroxil, cefaclor, cefixime, ceftibuten
ceph-	Cephalosporins (antibiotics)	cephalexin, cephapirin, cephradine
cort-	Corticosteroids (anti-inflammatory)	cortisone
rifa-	Antituberculars	rifamate, rifampin, rifapentine, rifater
sulf-	Sulfanilamides (antibiotics)	sulfadiazine, sulfamethoxazole, sulfasoxazole
-actone	Potassium-sparing diuretics	aldactone, spironolactone
-ane	General anesthetics	cyclohexane, ethane, fluorane
-ase	Thrombolytics (clot-busters)	eminase, retavase, streptokinase
-azole	Antifungals	butoconazole, econazole, fluconazole
-azosin	Alpha blockers (adrenergic antagonists)	doxazosin, prazosin, terazosin
-barbital	Barbiturates (sedative-hypnotics)	amobarbital, pentobarbital, secobarbital
-caine	Local anesthetics	bupivacaine, cocaine, lidocaine, xylocaine
-calci-	Calcium & vitamin D supplements	calciferol, calcitriol, ergocalciferol
-cillin	Penicillins	ampicillin, penicillin
-ciclovir	Antivirals	famciclovir, ganciclovir
-dazole	Nitroimidazole Antimicrobial	metronidazole
-dipine	Calcium channel blockers	amlodipine, felodipine, isradipine, nifedipine
-dronate	Biphosphonates	alendronate, etidronate, pamidronate, risedronate
-ergot-	Ergotamines (anti-migraine)	ergotamine, dihydroergotamine
-floxacin	Fluoroquinolones (antibiotics)	ciprofloxacin, gatifloxacin, levofloxacin
-ine	Stimulants	amphetamine, caffeine, terbutaline, theophylline
-lam	Benzodiazepines (anxiolytics)	alprazolam, midazolam
-lol	Beta blockers (adrenergic antagonists)	atenolol, propanolol, sotalol
-lone	Corticosteroids (anti-inflammatory)	methylprednisolone, prednisolone, triamcinolone
-micin	Aminoglycosides (antibiotics)	gentamicin

Medication Prefixes and Suffixes

Medication Prefixes and Suffixes

Prefix/Suffix	Class	Examples
-mycin	Aminoglycosides/Macrolides (antibiotics)	erythromycin, tobramycin, vancomycin
-navir	HIV/AIDS antivirals	amprenavir, indinavir, nelfinavir, ritonavir
-pam	Benzodiazepines (anxiolytics)	diazepam, lorazepam
-parin	Anticoagulant	enoxaparin
-prazole	Proton pump inhibitors (anti-ulcer)	lansoprazole, omeprazole, pantoprazole
-pril	ACE inhibitors (antihypertensives)	captopril, moexipril, quinapril
-profen	NSAIDS (anti-inflammatory)	fenoprofen, ibuprofen, ketoprofen
-quine	Antiparasitics	chloroquine, hydroxychloroquine
-sartan	Angiotensin-II receptor antagonists	candesartan, losartan, telmisartan, valsartan
-semide	Loop Diuretic	furosemide
-setron	5-HT3 receptor antagonists (antiemetics)	dolasetron, granisetron, ondansetron
-sone	Corticosteroids (anti-inflammatory)	cortisone, dexamethasone, prednisone
-statin	HMG-CoA Reductase inhibitor	rosuvastatin, atorvastatin, simvastatin
-stigmine	Cholinergics	neostigmine, physostigmine, pyridostigmine
-stine	Antineoplastics (anti-tumor)	carmustine, lomustine, vinblastine, vincristine
-terol	Bronchodilators	albuterol, bitolterol, levalbuterol, pirbuterol
-thiazide	Thiazide Diuretics	benzthiazide, hydrochlorothiazide
-tidine	H2 receptor antagonists (anti-ulcer)	cimetidine, famotidine, nizatidine, ranitidine
-triptan	Anti-migraines	naratripan, rizatriptan
-triptyline	Tricyclics (antidepressants)	amitriptyline, nortriptyline, protriptyline
-vir	Antivirals	abacivir, zanamivir
-vudine	HIV/AIDS antivirals	lamivudine, stavudine, zidovudine
-zolam	Benzodiazepines (anxiolytics)	alprazolam, midazolam
-zine	Phenothiazines (antipsychotics,antiemetics)	chlorpromazine, perphenazine, prochlorperazine
-zoline	Nasal decongestants	oxymetazoline, xylometazoline

Insulin Administration

Insulin Administration

TYPE	BRAND NAME	GENERIC NAME	ONSET	PEAK	DURATION
Rapid-Acting	NovoLog	Insulin aspart	15m	30-90m	3-5h
Rapid-Acting	Apidra	Insulin glulisine	15m	30-90m	3-5h
Rapid-Acting	Humalog	Insulin lispro	15m	30-90m	3-5h
Short-Acting	Humulin R	Regular	30-60m	2-4h	5-8h
Short-Acting	Novolin R	Regular	30-60m	2-4h	5-8h
Intermediate Acting	Humulin N	NPH	1-3h	8h	12-16h
Intermediate Acting	Novolin N	NPH	1-3h	8h	12-16h
Pre-Mixed NPH w/Regular	Humulin 70/30	70%NPH and 30% Reg	30-60m	varies	10-16h
Pre-Mixed NPH w/Regular	Novolin 70/30	70%NPH and 30% Reg	30-60m	varies	10-16h
Pre-Mixed NPH w/Regular	Humulin 50/50	50%NPH and 50% Reg	30-60m	varies	10-16h

Diabetic Ketoacidosis (DKA) Care

Results from the body breaking down cellular fat for energy which results in high levels of ketones. Ususally occurs in type I diabetics.

Care:

Correct fluid loss (fluid administration)
Correct hyperglycemia (insulin)
Correct electrolyte abnormalities
Correct ABG
Assess for infection or cause

HHNS Care

Results from a relative insulin deficiency. Blood sugar passes into the urine bringing water with it. The patient becomes very dehydrated. Occurs most often in type II diabetics.

Care:

Rehydration
Correct hyperglycemia (insulin)
Assess for underlying cause

Pharm Math Equations

Pharm Math Equations

$$\text{Drops per minute} = \frac{\text{Volume} * \text{Drip Factor}}{\text{Time (in minutes)}}$$

$$\text{Infusion time} = \frac{\text{Volume to be infused}}{\text{mL per hour}}$$

$$\text{Milliters per hour} = \frac{\text{Volume (mL)}}{\text{Hours}}$$

$$\text{Dosage} = \frac{\text{Desired Dose}}{\text{Available Dose}} * \text{Quantity}$$

1mL=1cc
1L=1000mL
1kg=2.2lbs
1tsp=5mL
1tbsp=15mL
1oz=30mL
12oz=360mL
1cup=8oz=240mL

PEDIATRIC PHARMACOLOGY

Carry out to the hundreths DO NOT round

Dosage based on mg/kg or BSA (body surface area)

Steps to Calculations:

Calculate daily dose ordered
Calculate low and high parameters
Compare dose to safe ranges

IM Injection Sites

IM Injection Sites

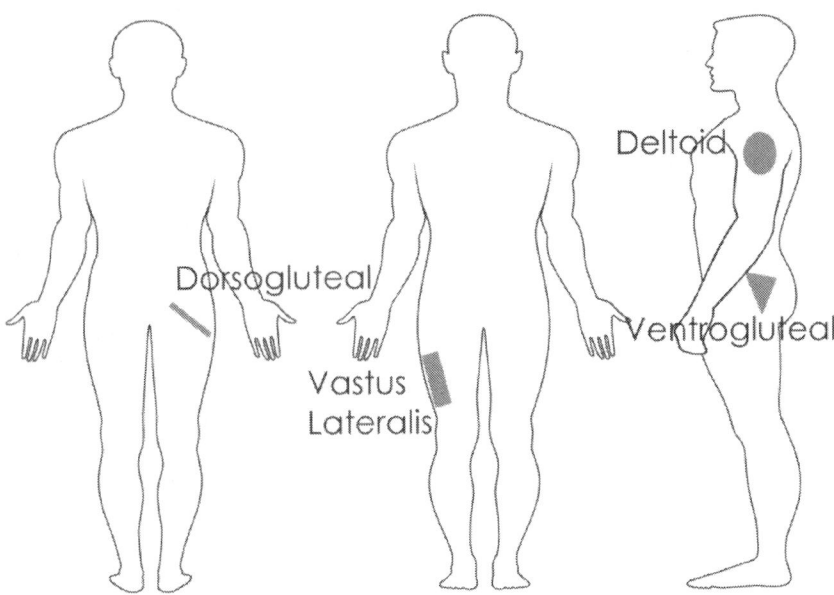

Vastus Lateralis:
  Lateral middle third of the thigh between the greater trochanter and knee.

Deltoid:
  2.5-5cm below the lower edge of the acromion process.

Ventrogluteal:
  Place palm of hand over greater trochanter forming a V with middle finger pointing toward iliac crest and index finger toward anterior superior liac spine.

Immunization Schedule

Immunization Schedule

Vaccine	BIRTH	**BABY (months)** 1	2	4	6	12	15	18	**CHILD (years)** 19-23	2-3	4-6
HepB	HepB	HepB	HepB		HepB	HepB	HepB				
RV			RV	RV	RV						
TDaP			TDaP	TDaP	TDaP						TDaP
Hib			Hib	Hib	Hib	Hib	Hib				
PCV			PCV	PCV	PCV	PCV	PCV				
IPV			IPV	IPV	IPV	IPV					IPV
Influenza										Yearly	
MMR						MMR	MMR				MMR
Varicella						Varicella	Varicella				Varicella
HepA								HepA	HepA		

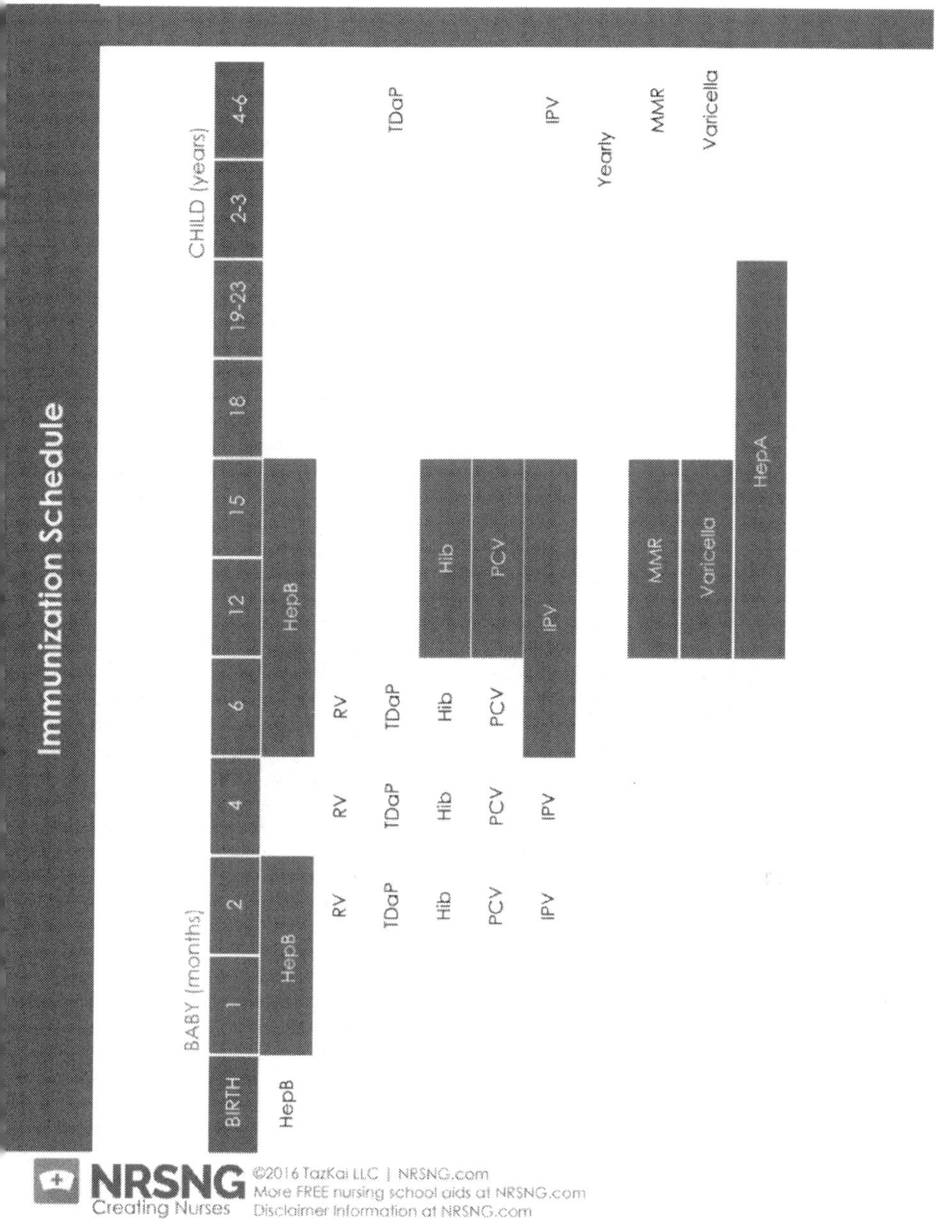

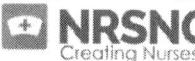

Pediatric BSA Burn Chart

Pediatric BSA Burn Chart

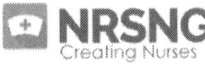

Based on Lund Browder Chart

AREA	BIRTH	AGE 1 YR	AGE 5 YR
A: 1/2 of Head	9 1/2	8 1/2	6 1/2
B: 1/2 of Thigh	2 3/4	3 1/4	4
C: 1/2 of Leg	2 1/2	2 1/2	2 3/4

AREA	AGE 10 YR	AGE 15 YR	ADULT
A: 1/2 of Head	5 1/2	4 1/2	3 1/2
B: 1/2 of Thigh	4 1/2	4 1/2	4 3/4
C: 1/2 of Leg	3	3 1/4	3 1/2

Fetal Circulation

Fetal Circulation

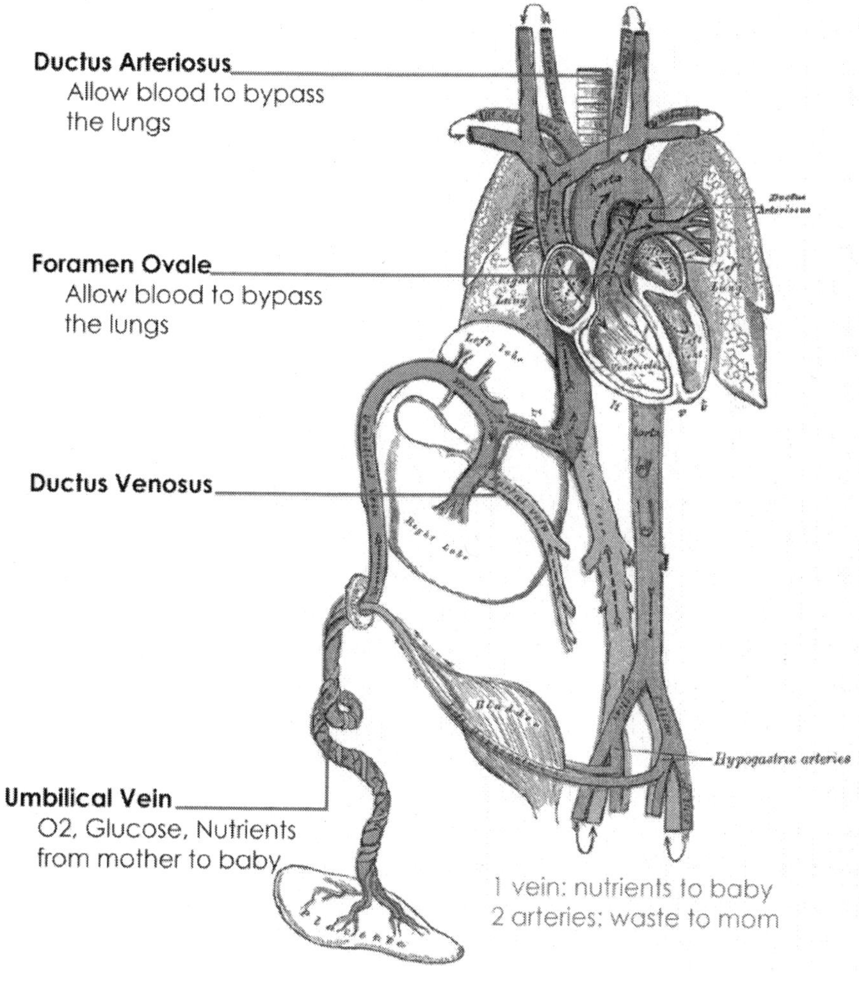
Ductus Arteriosus
Allow blood to bypass the lungs
Foramen Ovale
Allow blood to bypass the lungs
Ductus Venosus
Umbilical Vein
O2, Glucose, Nutrients from mother to baby
Hypogastric arteries
Bladder
1 vein: nutrients to baby
2 arteries: waste to mom

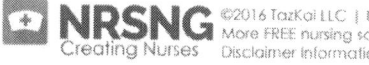

Newborn Assessment

Newborn Assessment

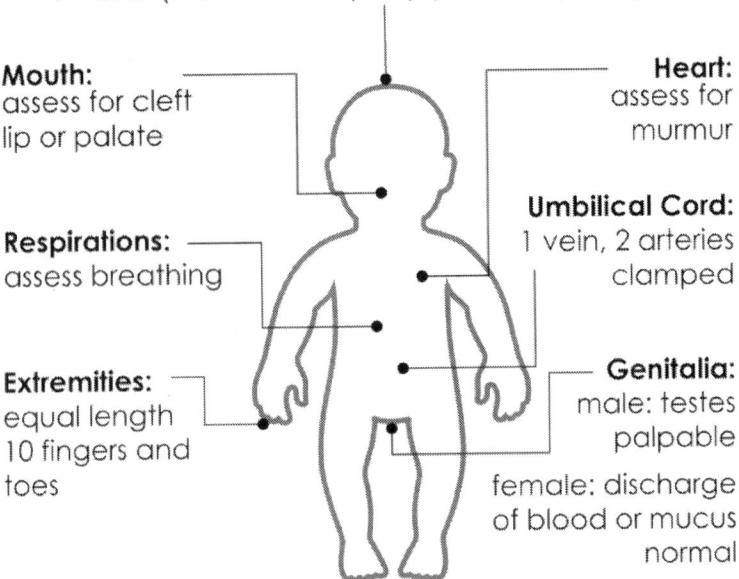

Appearance: pink, loud cry, well-flexed, full ROM

Fontanelles:
anterior (diamond-shaped), porterior (triangular)

Mouth: assess for cleft lip or palate

Heart: assess for murmur

Umbilical Cord: 1 vein, 2 arteries clamped

Respirations: assess breathing

Extremities: equal length 10 fingers and toes

Genitalia: male: testes palpable

female: discharge of blood or mucus normal

NEWBORN MEDS AND LABS

Vitamin K: prevent hemorrhage
Optic Antibiotic: prevent newborn blindness
PKU Level: within 24 hrs after feeding begins
Coombs' Test: if mother Rh-neg.
Immunizations: Hep-B can be given

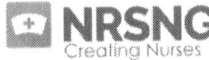

Nursing Mnemonics

Nursing Mnemonics

OB/PEDS

Cyanotic Defects

The 4 T's
Tetralogy of Fallot
Truncus Arteriosus
Transposition of the Great Vessels
Tricuspid Atresia

Episiotomy - Evaluation of Healing

REEDA
Redness
Edema
Eccymosis
Discharge
Approximation

Fetal Accelerations and Decelerations

VEAL CHOP
Variable - Cord Compression
Early - Head Compression
Accelerations - Okay
Late - Placental Insufficiency

Non-Stress Test

NNN
Non-reactive
Non-Stress is
Not-good

Severe Pre-Eclampsia Signs and Symptoms

HELLP
Hemolysis
Elevated
Liver Function tests
Low
Platelet count

Hypoxia - Signs and Symptoms

FINES
Feeding difficulty
Inspiratory stridor
Nares flares
Expiratory grunting
Sternal retractions

LABS

Hyperkalemia - Causes

MACHINE
Medications: ACE inhibitors, NSAIDS, K sparing diuretics
Acidosis: metabolic and respiratory
Cellular destruction: burns, injury, hemolysis
Hypoaldosteronism: Addisons
Intake: excess
Nephrons: renal failure
Excretion: impaired

Hyperkalemia-Management

KIND
Kayexalate
Insulin
Na HCO3
Diuretics

Hypernatremia-Causes

MODEL
Medications/Meals
Osmotic diuretics
Diabetes insipidus
Excessive water loss
Low water intake

Hypocalcemia-Signs/Symptoms

CATS
Convulsions
Arrhythmias
Tetany
Spasms and Stridor

Hyponatremia-Signs/Symptoms

SALT LOSS
Stupor/coma
Anorexia
Lethargy
Tendon reflexes decreased

Limp Muscles
Orthostatic hypotension
Seizures
Stomach cramping

PHARMACOLOGY

Beta 1 and Beta 2

Beta1: you have 1 heart
Beta2: you have 2 lungs

Bradycardia Drugs

IDEA
Isoproterenol
Dopamine
Epinephrine
Atropine Sulfate

Emergency Drugs

Drugs to LEAN on
Lidocaine
Epinephrine
Atropine Sulfate
Narcan

Steroid Side Effects

6 S's
Sugar: hyperglycemia
Soggy bones: osteoporosis
Sick: decreased immunity
Sad: depression
Salt: water and salt retention
Sex: decreased libido

Lidocaine Toxicity

Slurred speech
Altered central nervous system
Muscle twitching
Seizures

Diuretic Classes

Leak Over The CAN
Loop
Osmotics
Thiazide
Carbonic anhydrase inhibitors
Aldosterone inhibitors
Na channel blockers

Nursing Mnemonics

Nursing Mnemonics

MENTAL HEALTH

Anorexia - signs and symptoms

ANOREXIA
Amenorrhea
No organic factors accounts for weight loss
Obviously thin but feels FAT
Refusal to maintain normal body weight
Epigastric discomfort is common
X-symptoms (peculiar symptoms)
Intense fears of gaining weight
Always thinking of foods

Alcoholism-behavioral problems

5 D's
Denial
Dependency
Demanding
Destructive
Domineering

Alzheimer's Disease

5 As
Amnesia – loss of memories
Anomia – unable to recall names of everyday objects
Apraxia – unable to perform tasks of movement
Agnosia – inability to process sensory information
Aphasia – disruption with ability to communicate

MED SURG

Dyspnea

6 Ps
Pulmonary Bronchial Constriction
Possible Foreign Body
Pulmonary Embolus
Pneumothorax
Pump Failure
Pneumonia

Hyperglycemia vs Hypoglycemia

Hyper - hot/dry - sugar high
Hypo - cold/clammy - needs candy

MED SURG

Arterial Blood Gas Evaluation

ROME
Respiratory
Opposite
Metabolic
Equal

Pulmonary Edema - treatment

MAD DOG
Morphine – causes vasodilation resulting in decreased BP
Aminophylline – relaxes airways to make breathing easier
Digitalis – improve heart function in pulmonary edema

Diuretics (Lasix) – pull excess fluid off
Oxygen – improve oxygenation
Gases (Blood Gases ABGs) – asses respiratory status

Hypoxia - signs/symptoms

RAT BED
Early Hypoxia:
Restlessness
Anxiety
Tachycardia/Tachypnea

Late Hypoxia:
Bradycardia
Extreme Restlessness
Dyspnea

Asthma - management

ASTHMA
Adrenergic (Albuterol)
Steroids
Theophylline
Hydration (IV)
Mask (Oxygen)
Antibiotics

Pupillary reaction

PERRLA
Pupils
Equally
Round and
Reactive to
Light and
Accommodate

MED SURG

Moles - malignant assessment

ABCD's
Asymmetry--is the mole irregular in shape?
Border--is the border irregular, notched, or poorly defined?
Color--does the color vary (for example, between shades of brown, red, white, blue, or black)?
Diameter--is the diameter more than 6 mm?

Hypoglycemia-signs/symptoms

TIRED
Tachycardia
Irritability
Restless
Excessive Hunger
Diaphoresis/ Depression
Sulfate

Cardiac Blood Flow

Toilet Paper My A''
Tricuspid
Pulmonic
Mitrial
Aortic

Cranial Nerves

Oh Oh Oh To Touch And Feel Very Good Velvet AH!
Olfactory
Optic
Oculomotor
Trochlear
Trigeminal
Abducens
Facial
Vestibulocochlear
Glossopharyngeal
Vagus
Accessory
Hypoglossal

Hypertension - complications

4 C's
Coronary Artery Disease
Coronary Rheumatic Fever
Congestive Heart Failure
Cerebral Vascular Accident

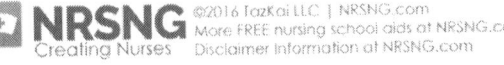

Head to Toe Assessment Checklist

Recommended order for head to toe assessment-not intended to be a complete assessment guide.

- General Assessment
- Body Structure/Mobility
- Behavior
- Health History
- Vital Signs
  - Height Weight
  - Pulse Rate
  - Respirations
  - Temperature
  - Blood Pressure
  - Pain
- Integumentary
  - Inspect: color, moisture, hair, rashes, lesions, pallor, edema
  - Palpate: temperature, turgor, lesions, edema, texture
- Scalp
  - Inspect: shape, symmetry
  - Palpate: tenderness, deformity
- Nails
  - Inspect: shape, color
  - Palpate: capillary refill
- Head
  - Inspect: symmetry, shape, size, uniformity
- Neck
  - Inspect: symmetry, lesions, scars
  - Palpate: tenderness, lymph nodes, thyroid gland, TMJ
- Eyes
  - Inspect: interior and exterior, visual fields, acuity, reflexes
- Ears
  - Inspect: color, shape, symmetry, interior inspection
  - Palpate: tenderness, deformity
- Nose
  - Inspect: shape, symmetry, interior inspection
  - Palpate: frontal sinus, maxillary sinuses
- Mouth and Throat
  - Inspect: exterior and interior
- Thorax and Lungs (anterior and posterior)
  - Inspection: respiration quality, symmetry, deformity, tracheal location
  - Palpation: tenderness, fremitus, chest expansion
  - Percussion: percussive tones, diaphragmatic excursion
  - Auscultation: breath sounds and quality
- Heart and Great Vessels
  - Inspection: jugular venous pulse
  - Palpate: pulses, PMI
  - Auscultate: heart sounds (bell and diaphragm)

- Peripheral Vascular System
  - Inspect: color, edema
  - Palpate: temperature, edema
- Abdomen
  - Inspect: discomfort, uniformity, color, symmetry, scars, hernia, peristalsis, pulsations
  - Auscultate: bowel sounds, bruits
  - Percussion: four quadrants, liver, spleen, renal tenderness
  - Palpation: light to deep, liver, spleen, aorta, rebound tenderness, fluid wave
- Musculoskeletal
  - Inspection: asymmetry, deformity, atrophy
  - Palpation: major joints, tenderness, deformity, range of motion
- Neurological
  - Inspect: mental status (health history), cranial nerves, coordination, movement, senses
  - Palpate: motor strength, muscle tone, reflexes, senses
- Genitourinary
  - Inspect: general appearance, lesions, scars
  - Palpate: breast exam, testicular exam, prostate exam, vaginal exam, Pap smear
- Lymphatic
  - Palpate: assess lymph node locations

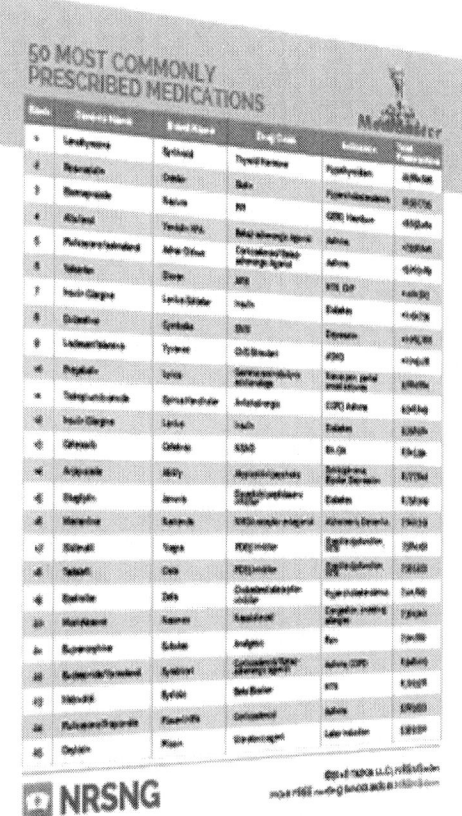

Made in the USA
Lexington, KY
09 March 2017